A Battle With Covid-19

How I Healed Myself

Diondra Flowers

ISBN- 978-1-71683-967-2

Printed in the United States of America

My heart goes out to everyone who has lost someone they love to this virus and to those who are currently suffering.

We are all in this together.

PREFACE

The Content is not intended to be a substitute for professional medical advice, diagnosis, or treatment. Always see the advice of your physician or other qualified health providers with any questions you may have regarding a medical condition. Never disregard professional medical advice or delay in seeking it because of something you may have read within this book.

 If you think you may have a medical emergency, call your doctor, go to the nearest emergency room, or call 911 immediately.

INTRODUCTION

The world changed unexpectedly in the early part of 2020. Millions of people were stricken by the deadly Covid-19 virus, with hundreds of thousands dying. A Battle with Covid-19 An intimate 30 Day Journal is the harrowing story of one woman's struggle to not only stay alive, but to keep her three children alive as well. How I Healed Myself is a look at what I did to fight back and defy the odds I was given. I went to the hospital three times each time feeling worse than when I had arrived and to make matters worse doctors had no clue what was wrong with me. I did dozens of blood tests, CAT scans, and took several cocktails the made everything I was dealing with in my body 10x worse. A drive thru testing center was made available and I went only to be confronted with my worst fears. This book is insight on what I did when I made the decision to stay home and treat myself after being told I needed to be hospitalized again. Not only was I sick but my 3 children were as well. I did a lot of research and this book is a list of everything that helped me and my children. I hope it will help you as well.

DETOX

Detox Water

1-inch Ginger Root

1 Lemon

1 tsp Turmeric

1-gallon Alkaline Water

Juice half of the lemon and thinly slice the other half. Cut off I inch of the ginger root and slice it thin. Add both to the water also add the teaspoon of turmeric and shake well. I drink at room temperature, but some may prefer it to be cold.

Benefits

- o <u>Ginger</u>: natural pain reliever, anti-inflammatory, settle an upset stomach, and curb nausea
- o <u>Lemon</u>: promotes hydration, good source for vitamin C, limit the duration of the common cold, protects cells from free radicals, and aid in digestion
- o <u>Turmeric</u>: helps with the release of stress hormones, good for joints and joint pain, and good for digestion
- o <u>Alkaline Water</u>: removes heavy metals from the body, hydrates the body and improves water absorption, improves overall digestion, improves and relieves pain in muscles and joints, and promotes and increases energy.

I drank at least one 16oz glass/bottle of this every day. Some days I would sip it throughout the day others I would drink it in the morning. I also increased the amount I drank as I was able to keep down more. One of the most important parts of recovery is to stay hydrated. I used this particular combination to ease my nausea, boost my immune system, increase oxygen flow and hydrate. I wasn't able to keep anything down. I was trying to remedy my headache which I knew was in part due to being dehydrated and it did work. After the first day I could tell the difference.

It is absolutely essential for you to start a hydration regimen as early as you can. Not being hydrated left me with a headache, feeling faint, muscle aches and also weak.

NUTRIENTS

V8 Fusion

My Favs

- Healthy Greens
- Peach Mango
- Pomegranate Blueberry
- Strawberry Banana
- Acai Mixed Berry

Benefits

Most give you a serving of fruit and a serving of vegetables.

 I would suggest drinking one full size bottle a day which equals out to about 6 servings. I sipped this throughout the as kind of a meal replacement when I was not able to hold down any solids. Your body still needs its vitamins and nutrients. The good thing about this is it tastes like fruit juice and kids love it also. My kids drink this all the time anyway so that they can get all of their servings of fruit and veggies. With picky eaters this is a life saver. Once I added this, I could feel some of my energy coming back.

HYDRATE

Alkaline Water

Benefits

- Boosts Immune System
- Nurtures healthy blood cells
- Promotes strong muscles, joints and bones
- Increases energy through the power of hydrogen
- Helps recover after exercise or trauma and eases the aches and pains of muscles and joints
- Promotes better sleep
- Flushes out toxins and removes heavy metals
- Fights free radicals Hydrates by penetrating at a cellular level

- o Elevates oxygen levels
- o Delivers nutrients to the cells

I put this in my detox and drank this whenever I was vomiting. My goal was to continue to hydrate my body and replenish what was lost as quickly as I could.

I cannot express how important this was. If you are anything like me then you will be losing a lot of your fluids and since your body is made up of mostly water this is necessary. I chose Alkaline water for all of the added benefits.

VITAMINS

NutraBurst (Buy Here)

https://retail.totallifechanges.com/Flowerpoweroflove

Benefits

- o Great multivitamin
- o 98% absorption into the blood stream
- o Increase of energy
- o 72 Minerals
- o 18 Amino Acids
- o 10 Vitamin Extracts
- o 22 Phytonutrients
- o 13 Whole Food Greens
- o 12 Different Healthy Herbs

I added orange juice for taste. It does not have an appealing taste but an improvement from the earlier version. There is a hint of fruit, but it absolutely tastes like its contents. My regimen was to take this every morning. It is a liquid vitamin, so the absorption process is easier and more efficient. After the first day I did notice and improvement but by the third day there were definite signs that this was helping me out. It gave me the energy I needed to attempt to play with my children.

LUNG STRENGTH

Breathing Exercises

- <u>Blowing Up Balloons</u>
  - o I blew up a total of 3 balloons each time.
- <u>Diaphragmatic Breathing</u>
  - o Relax shoulders and sit back or lie down Place one hand on your belly and one on your chest
  - o Inhale through your nose for 2 seconds feeling the air move into your abdomen Your stomach should move more than your chest
  - o Breathe out for 2 seconds through pursed lips while pressing on your belly.

- <u>Hold Your Breath</u>
  - In through your nose
  - Hold as long as you can
  - Out through your mouth.

You do not have to do these back to back. I spread them out throughout the day. I actually made it into a game with my kids. You will have to push yourself a little. If you feel uncomfort or like you are in distress, please stop and contact your physician. This was a lifesaver for me. In the beginning it did hurt to breathe in deeply so much so that I avoided it for at least 3 days but felt like an eternity. After getting through the first few days it became easier. Please be advised this will tire you out. If you feel lightheaded, fatigued or extreme exhaustion stop and try again later.

ACHES AND PAINS

Stretching

Benefits

- o Increases Circulation
- o You stimulate blood to the muscles
- o Supplies muscles with the oxygen and essential nutrients
- o Carries waste materials from the muscle
- o Lowers stress levels Relieves physical tension
- o Gets a healthy supply of blood to the brain
- o Reduces pain
- o Eases soreness

Simple stretches are enough to see a difference. I stretched with my children every morning and every night. I made a point to stretch all the areas that were sore. This will be uncomfortable in the beginning but after the 2nd day it will feel better. I also recommend that you soak in a hot bath and inhale the steam while you are in there. The body aches were the least of my worries, but they were present. A few minutes a day in combination with the other things on the list ceased my muscle spasms and eased the aches.

REACT

Probiotics

Benefits

- o Live Micro Organisms
- o Gut Health
- o Treat Diarrhea
- o Heart Health
- o Boost Immune System

I put a probiotic mix into my kids' juice and had them drink it daily. They had been doing this before Covid-19 and I just kept it going. This could be one of the main reasons that their symptoms were so mild. You will definitely notice the difference after the 2nd or third use. This did not have a strong taste. I like to mix things with orange juice but I mixed my kids with the V8 Fusion and they couldn't tell the difference. I purchased my packets online.

I can honestly say that this does have some pretty impressive benefits.

MEDICINES

Benadryl & Mucinex DM

- Benadryl
  - o Treats nausea, vomiting and dizziness
- Mucinex DM
  - o Loosens mucus and phlegm and thins out bronchial secretions

I understand that some people only feel comfortable if meds are added and this was 2 that I briefly tried, and my mother took continuously that gave her results.

The Benadryl was to alleviate the dizziness, nausea and vomiting, it was also a help with the headache. The Mucinex will loosen all mucus. If you do have a cough this will aid in making it more productive. My cough was more so due to the shortness of breath.

REGROUP

Prayer/Meditation

Whichever you choose or both is fine.

Benefits

- o Peace of mind
- o Lower Stress
- o Decrease Anxiety
- o Decrease Depression
- o Increase Emotional Stability

Whether you enjoy talking or listening you can benefit from the healing properties of peace of mind. I found that it continues to give you hope. Taking a moment whenever things seem hard or you are feeling overwhelmed will have significant results. Regardless of where your faith lies, we all want peace and positive energy. I partook of both meditation, prayer and my own personal chants. It definitely put me in a better headspace and allowed me to clear my mind in that moment so that I could keep my sanity. With so many worries and fears this was a necessary task.

REJUVENATE

Sleep

This may be one of the most important on the list.

The average adult needs 7 to 9 hours of sleep.

Benefits

- o Reduces Stress
- o Increases Heart Health
- o Boosts Immune System & Function
- o Essential for Brain Function
- o Repair & Restore Organ System
- o Repair Muscles

I was always very fatigued but extreme fatigue would hit and I could not keep my eyes open. Sleep as much and as often as you can. If you feel the need to rest and you can please do so. As a mother of 3 kids I was not able to sleep as much as I should have but I felt a little better after waking from a lengthy sleep session.

INSPIRATION

- ❖ Whatever you enjoy,
- ❖ Whatever gives you hope.
- ❖ Whatever gives you strength
- ❖ Whatever encourages.
- ❖ Whatever makes you want to fight.
- ❖ Whatever gives you positive energy.

My inspiration was my children. I knew I had to try to muster up whatever strength I had left to fight for them. I used my fears to work for me. I told myself I could not fail. I allowed their laughter to motivate me. I let their love lift me into a positive mindset when I would get discouraged. Find who or what you enjoy and use that as your reason to fight, your reason to keep going, your reason to not give up.

AFTERWORD

Looking back on this short journey going through it seemed like it was forever. During the beginning stages it was physically and emotionally draining, I could literally feel death on me. I was terrified, more so for my children than for myself. I did not want them to find me unresponsive or have to go through life without a me to love and watch over them. Most people have been spreading that this is like the flu, but it is not! I have had the flu, and this is by far different.

 In the beginning it came on with what I thought was a headache which grew into a migraine and then to the worst head pain I had ever felt in my life. The headache was accompanied by vomiting, nausea, dizziness and a feeling of being lightheaded. The feeling is continuous opening my eyes, turning my head, getting up and just about anything that required movement. Its mad normal task like going to the bathroom a hazard because not only did I feel horrible, but I was unsteady and passed out quite a few times. This was so bad I did not really care about the other symptoms until I was able to get this under control. Add to the mix shortness of breath! This was the stage where I felt I could possibly die. Fever and chills were frequent, and I could not keep anything down, not to mention I was delirious most of the time.

Once those symptoms set in, I noticed that not only could I not taste or smell anything, but my mouth was coated in the most horrible taste ever. It literally causes even water to taste poisonous. As you would expect eating was not really an option.

Through the entire ordeal I was in fear. Fear for my children. Fear for my life. Fear this life would be permanent.

I still am not sure if there will be any lasting damage to our bodies and I pray not.

The items that I listed in this book absolutely helped pull me from the depths in which I thought there was no return. If you choose to follow this, please start at the earliest signs

BOOKS IN THIS SERIES

A Battle with Covid-19

This series is an up-close and personal look at the journey battling the novel coronavirus that is currently plaguing the world.

A Battle with COvid-19 A 30 Day Intimate Journal This is an inside look at what I went through physically, mentally and emotionally.

Covid-19 We Fight Together This is a children's book that my 10-year-old daughter wanted to write to give a look at it for children.

A Battle with Covid-19 How I Healed Myself This is a detailed look at what I did to recover from almost being hospitalized.

www.ingramcontent.com/pod-product-compliance
Lightning Source LLC
Chambersburg PA
CBHW061325250726

48657CB00003B/1052